9/25/03

Dear Dirk,

I'm looking forward to working with you in 2004 to customize my <u>Superior Service</u> program for your affiliate. I'm confident the tools & techniques provided will increase your customers' loyalty!

Warmly,
Patti Hathaway, CSP

Proverbs 12:18

Banking Secrets for Customer Loyalty: Handling Customer Problems

by Patti Hathaway, CSP
Editor: Tim Polk
Cartoonist: Dom Rinaldo
Back cover photo by Brian T. Shindle/Creative Moments

Published by:

Destination Publications
1016 Woodglen Road
Westerville, Ohio 43081-3236 U.S.A.

Printed in the United States of America

Library of Congress Cataloging-in-Publication Data
Hathaway, Patti

Banking Secrets for Customer Loyalty: Handling Customer Problems/ by Patti Hathaway

ISBN 0-9678731-6-9 (pbk.)
Library of Congress Card Number: 2002093251

Banking Secrets

for Customer Loyalty

Handling
Customer
Problems

Patti Hathaway, CSP

 Destination Publications,
Westerville, Ohio

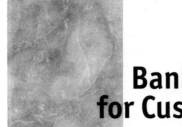

Banking Secrets for Customer Loyalty:

Handling Customer Problems

Table of Contents

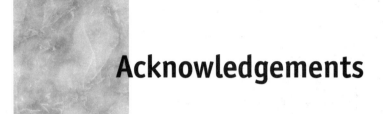

Acknowledgements

A heartfelt thanks to my husband and business partner Jim for managing the business so I can do what I do best and for being my biggest fan and supporter.

A special acknowledgement to those who provided me with their technical assistance: Tim Polk, editor; Dom Rinaldo, cartoonist; Gary Hoffman, typesetter and cover designer; and Claudia Earlenbach, transcriptionist.

Thanks to those of you who have reviewed and endorsed my book: Robert K. Healey, Jr., R. Daniel Sadlier, and Max Wells. To the following people I want to extend my special thanks for allowing me to use their letters and/or quotes throughout my book: Cindy Bush, Barbara Carmen, Michael Ferrell, Roger Furrer, Andrew Rosen, Douglas Singer, Max Wells, and Nancy Zikmanis. Thanks also to those authors whose books I read and quoted: The Gallup Management Journal; Jeffrey Gitomer, CSP; and Manuel J. Smith, Ph.D.

Most importantly, I would like to thank all the people who have attended my keynotes and seminars over the years and who have expanded my views on customer loyalty in banks. Many of your quotes and examples are included in my book.

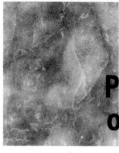

Prepaying a Funeral or Precipitating It?

He was a 59-year-old man who lived a modest life, but he was ill with heart problems. His greatest concern in life was that he would die and not be able to pay for his funeral expenses. However, he was expecting a small inheritance from his aunt. One day he opened his mail and was shocked to discover that $183,516 had been added to his bank account. He never knew his aunt was that wealthy and didn't quite believe it. He called up his bank. The Customer Service Representative who answered the phone checked the computer system and said, "Yes, $183,516.11 has been added to your account." He was still not convinced. He had one sibling, a sister. He and his sister went down to the branch office where he typically did his banking to make sure the money was his before he began spending it. Again, the bank confirmed that the money was indeed his.

He went immediately to the funeral home. He prepaid his funeral expenses and bought himself a steel gray casket. He was feeling very good about that purchase because he didn't want to leave his sister with any burdens. Then he gave $18,000 to his sister and her two children. He also bought a used van.

Several weeks later however, the FBI swooped in on him and arrested him for bank fraud. He spent three weeks in jail while the attorneys wrangled back and forth. He finally was released from jail on bail. The day after he was released from jail, he and a friend were getting into his used van (which he thought he had paid for legitimately) when he suffered a stroke. His friend quickly called 9-1-1. The emergency squad

---

* The story is true. Names have been changed.

BANKING SECRETS
═══•COM═══

rushed him to the hospital. Two days later he died of a heart attack. Mr. Randolph's sister believes that the bank killed her brother. *

If I had been one of your customers who read this article in our local major metropolitan newspaper about your bank, and then came into your banking center and said, "I know your bank charges a lot of fees, but this is ridiculous – Are you now killing people?" What would you have said to me – a slightly irate, and potentially challenging, customer?

First, let me tell you the rest of the opening story as it actually happened to a banking client of mine: Mr. Clyde Randolph had a very lengthy white-collar criminal record not reported in the newspaper. In fact, much of his criminal history had to do with bank fraud. The error? Not the bank's. The wire transfer company transferred money into Mr. Randolph's account by mistake. However, the bank ended up being the "bad guy" by having to pursue legal action to get the money back. Here is the quandary for you: If this had been your bank, your customers would probably never learn the rest of the story. Yet you will need to handle the customers who come in and ask you about the reported incident. How do you typically handle customers who have problems with your bank?

How do you handle the not-so-happy or even angry customers who call you or visit your branch? What we're going to talk about in this book is *how* to handle the problem situations and angry customers you encounter.

So What Makes Exceptional Customer Service?

The type of customer service you deliver has two dimensions. One dimension involves the **System** side of what you do. The system side includes all the procedures your bank has in place, including its rules, regulations, and fees. It is how bank employees work together to serve customers. The opening story involves a system problem. The wire transfer company's *system* made several errors which the bank had to clean up, and the partial truth got reported in the local newspaper.

The **Style** dimension is our traditional view of customer service. It's your attitude. It's how you answer the phones. It's how you greet people. It's how you handle upset customers. It's everything that you personally do with your customers day in and day out.

There are four different ways you can combine these two dimensions.

Iceberg Service

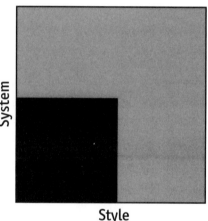

Both the style and system dimensions in the Iceberg service model are low. If you provide this type of service, you may expect the following results: Customers are closing their accounts. A CSR states: "It's not my fault, it's the bank's fault." Customers complain: "We aren't paying $8 for you to cash our check. That's ridiculous!" "You don't have enough help here." " I'm a senior citizen, why do I have to pay for money orders and official checks?" "I've been banking with you for 22 years: why do you still ask to see my driver's license?"

Iceberg Service means that your bank employees will only see the tip of the iceberg. Not seen beneath the semi-calm customer waters is the huge bolder ready to explode against your bank or you. The message to the customer simply is, *"We don't really care about you or the bank."* If the customer wants to close their account, you give them the paperwork. If the customer wants to open an account, you grudingly help them. "What Mr. Customer? You have a complaint? What are you complaining to me for? Do I look like I can do anything here?"

Here are several actual customer letters involving *Iceberg*- style service. When I provide you with negative examples, I will not disclose the actual bank involved. However, for the positive letters and examples, I'll provide the name of the bank and where the incident occurred.

"Three months ago, I spent most of Saturday morning discussing my banking needs with so-and-so at ABC Bank. She assured me that ABC Bank could certainly accommodate all my needs. I opened an interest-bearing checking account. At the time, I made her aware that I am here on an H1B visa and that my wife is not allowed to have a Social Security number with her H4 visa. We both filled in all the necessary paperwork, and she assured us everything was in order. After a month passed, however, we became concerned that we had not received our debit cards. I called the bank." (The first person that he had initially talked with was now no longer with that branch so now he talked to a second person.)

After explaining our situation, this employee investigated and much to our dismay informed us that not only was my wife not in the system but the signature card that she had signed could not be located. She assured us that all that would need to be required was to get another copy of my wife's signature and my authorization." [On arrival at the branch, the second person was not available so now the customer is referred to a third person.]

After explaining our situation to her, to our surprise, this employee immediately stated that my wife could not be added to the checking account as a co-signatory since she does not have a Social Security number. She said this was company policy. This was the first time anyone had said that it would be a problem. Not once in our previous contacts with your bank had anyone mentioned this policy. In fact, we had not only received

the checks, my wife had been signing them for three months.

Much to our dismay, this employee offered no other options and did not seem concerned that our paperwork had been misplaced. Rather, she made the original person the scapegoat, informing us that she didn't know what she was doing. Words cannot express how unsafe we felt with our personal and private information having being lost by your branch or being informed that your banking representative was incompetent. We insisted that the employee investigate this matter further. And when she refused us any further assistance, we asked to speak to the manager. Her only offer was that we call back on Monday to speak with the bank manager.

After further insistence on our part, she responded by asking us to leave, and when we refused, called the police department to have our two young daughters and us escorted out of the building. The police came and, unlike this employee, acted very professionally. They realized that my family posed no threat to your bank and, after explaining the situation, allowed us to stay and finish our business.

Not once did we receive an apology from this employee for our inconvenience. Not once did we feel any concern from her for having had our personal information lost by her branch and how insecure that made us feel. Not once did we feel that she had any concern about us as customers. Rather, we felt threatened. We felt as though we were criminals not customers. My young daughters are still deeply affected by the police pulling their mommy and daddy aside for questioning.

Is this the example of customer service that I've heard so much about at ABC Bank? Is this what your advertising means? I'm very upset by this sad episode, but even more importantly concerned about my personal information having been lost. I feel your bank has compromised my security.

Understandably, as my last business with this employee, I closed my checking account with ABC, and I'm initiating having my car loan transferred to another bank."

In this situation, clearly the bank had *system* problems in that employees at the same banking center understood banking policies differently and they couldn't locate the signature card among other issues. Plus, their *style* was to blame the customer for the problem and try to throw them out of the bank. Not actions or attitudes that are going to endear you to your customers!

This next letter is actually a lengthy handwritten statement on the closed account survey. In this particular case, several things have gone wrong. The bank had sent this particular family three different debit cards, all which were incorrect. Their son's name was misspelled on the savings account. In their words, here is the reason why they closed their account:

> *"The final straw came when we went to pull money out of the ATM. It was closed for repairs. We went to a second ATM for ABC Bank. It was also shut down. We finally went to another bank's ATM and were charged the fee of $1.50. It was 9:30 p.m. at night. We didn't feel like we should have to keep driving around.*
>
> *When we arrived home, we called the 800 (customer service) number and told them both ATM machines in this particular part of the city were not working, and we felt we should not be charged the fee from ABC Bank for using another bank. We were told they would notify the problems of the ATM in order to get them fixed, but we needed to contact the branch in order to reverse the charges of using another ATM. Next morning, we called the branch. They said they would not reverse the charges. I explained that we had gone to another ABC Bank ATM and it was not in service either. She then told us, 'There*

are other ATMs in the area.' I told her they were not that close.
She said that did not matter.

I then called the 800 number to complain about this mat-
ter. They told me there was nothing they could do. Both women
were not nice or helpful. In fact, they acted put out for having
to take my complaint. It made me feel we were not valued as
customers. I now bank with a company who meets these needs.
I feel ABC Bank does a poor job of customer service and have
advised others of this. I'll never bank with your company
again!"

This bank gave up a customer for a $1.50 fee reversal when it was the bank's fault that two of their ATM's were closed for repairs. Three different people were contacted by the customer and all three blamed the customer for the problem. How easy and inexpensive it would have been for any of those employees to simply reverse the charges and save the customer.

Here's what you need to know about Iceberg Service and the "we don't care" attitude: customers get angry. Jeffrey Gitomer, author of the book *Customer Satisfaction is Worthless, Customer Loyalty is Priceless**, discovered from research that:

- If you have a customer who leaves angry, 91 percent of them will never return.

- And 96 percent won't tell you the real reason they left.

To me, this high percent isn't surprising. In all the training that I have developed for banks, I have read many closed account surveys – those little cards that get sent out and returned when a customer closes their account. Most surveys have no comments on them – the customers just don't want to bother telling you why they left your bank. Here's the critical part of the research:

* Reprinted with permission from *Customer Satisfaction is Worthless, Customer Loyalty is Priceless* by Jeffrey Gitomer, BuyGitomer, Inc. www.gitomer.com

- 80 percent of angry customers will do business with you again **IF** their problem is handled quickly and to their complete satisfaction.

Our natural tendency as human beings if we have someone standing in front of us or calling us on the phone who says, "I've got a problem," is to think, "Oh no, not another angry customer! You know how many I've already had today? I don't get paid enough. Where's the manager?" We can't help but think, "Oh, I just don't want to deal with this person." We want to plug our ears and pass that person on to someone else to handle the problem.

You need to change your perspective right now! The next time you have a customer who says, "I've got a complaint" or "I have a problem,"

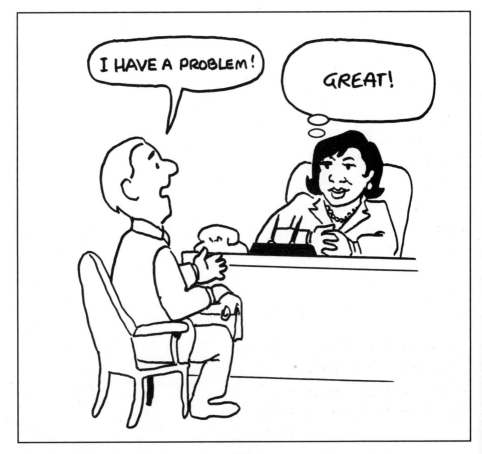

I want you to think in your head, "Great! I'm going to solve this problem and they're going to be back." That's what you need to be thinking and acting on! You must be committed to saving your customers!

What's scary to me is that many banks are closing almost as many accounts as they are opening. If your bank's emphasis is only on sales and not on servicing the customers, you basically are pouring your new accounts into a bank bucket with huge holes that are draining existing accounts out underneath. Customer service is about keeping the customer's money in your bank, not the on-going boom and bust of replacing lost customers with new customers. Keep in mind that customers are your paycheck.

How many of you have personally experienced lousy customer service? How many years have you been telling stories about that place? All your life, right? Every single chance you get to tell that story, you will tell about that horrible mechanic, travel agency, airline, hotel, restaurant, dry cleaners. It doesn't matter. We tell stories to everybody.

The question is: what stories are your banking customers telling about you? Do you notice I said, "You"? We are not talking about your bank, because YOU are the bank to your customers. We can fault the bank's systems, but in reality we are talking about your style and how you handle the problems your customer has with your bank. If your customer could describe the kind of service you give, what would they be saying about you?

The Wrong Way

Here is the nastiest letter I've ever read in all the time I've conducted customer service training. This actual letter is from a customer who is obviously very, very angry about the service her bank provided. Here is her story. This is written, by the way, in September.

"If we improve customer retention by 1% we will increase profits $1.1 million. That translates into saving one account per banking center per month."

Andrew S. Rosen,
Vice President & Deposit Product Manager
Fifth Third Bank

"For the second time since July 23, I am writing because you people do not get my address straight and are not sending my statements for 123456 and 789234. I have not had a savings account statement reach me since June 28. I have not received my checking account statement since July 27. I want you to send them and I want you to find my cancelled checks and send them too, now.

I'm a busy medical doctor and resident and neurologist at XYZ Medical Center who moved to this area a few months ago. I've dealt with many financial institutions in my life but have never yet dealt with one with a more amazing incapacity for customer service than ABC Bank. What do you have working for you – trained monkeys?

Every time I call your office about this, and it's been about four times, I'm informed that you still don't have my correct address on record. It comes out with a little variation every time. Now, if you were plumbers or sewer inspectors, it would not be so unexpected. However, you're a bank and you're supposed to have literate and numerate people working for you. Tell me, have you singled me out to victimize because I looked like a fun person to screw over? Or are you an equal opportunity and screw over all your customers?

Your staff sure feels sorry for themselves. Every time I call to complain, I get treated in a verbal manner as though I'm giving you people a hard time rather than the other way around. I spoke with a rude young person named so-and-so at the such-and-such an office today who has now become the fourth or fifth person to give me this routine. Disgusted with his whiney phone manners, I asked that he have the branch manager phone me.

Here are my demands... [She wants her statements, cancelled checks, a letter of apology, and she wants it all done by a certain date]

If you don't do these things, then I assure you, you have not heard the last from me. I'll contact the FDIC. I'll contact my attorney. Then I'll contact the press. I'll make your bank pay with public embarrassment for the time you're stealing from me, the time it takes me to write complaint letters like these, the time that I subtract from my studies and medical training. You see customers as nuisances rather than as your patrons. You see yourselves as doing the public some kind of big favor to let us invest money with you. Well, I'll tell you how I see you. You are nothing but a bunch of slovenly, hateful, uncaring, and incompetent people, the kind who compromise the cow patties in the pasture of life."

Angry customers will make you pay. However, they can also be beneficial. When someone has a complaint, that complaint is a gift. It's a gift for you to do something to help that person and to save their business for your bank.

Do you know how to correct/change the address of your customers at your bank? This is not an uncommon problem, particularly in very large banks. Your customers worry that someone will get unauthorized access to their accounts. They get so aggravated with the unreliability of the situation that they may eventually consider switching banks if the problem continues to be uncorrected.

Many banks have a master address base at the corporate headquarters, as well as addresses that must be changed at the local branch. All must be updated as some account information is sent from different departments and locations. Your key to customer success is knowing the right resources and owning the customer's problem.

Think about it: If you had a family member or friend who just moved into the area and now they need to find a new bank, would you recommend the bank you work for?

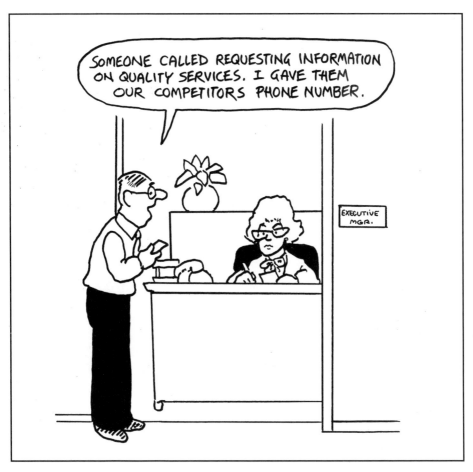

If you cannot, without hesitation, absolutely recommend your bank to your friends and family members, then something has to change. A good place to start is reading this book. Your bank must change how you deliver service so that you can, in fact, recommend your bank to other people.

The Right Way

It all began when one of the doctors at the Medical Center came in saying he was "very upset." It turned out that a replacement credit card was mailed to an old address in his

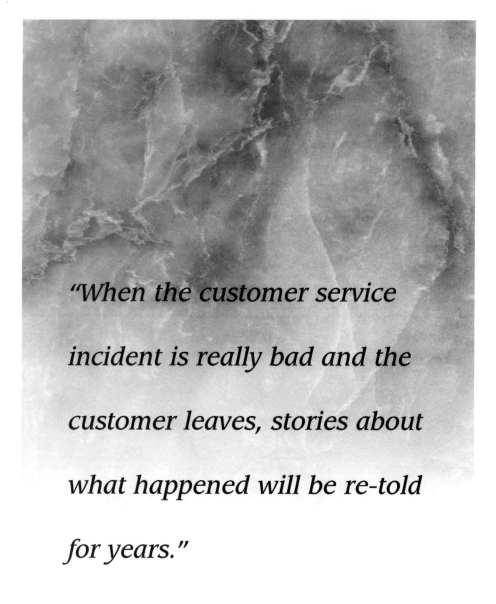

"When the customer service incident is really bad and the customer leaves, stories about what happened will be re-told for years."

Jeffrey Gitomer,
author of *Customer Satisfaction is Worthless,*
Customer Loyalty is Priceless

condo complex. *The last time he had gone to his branch (not ours) to update his address (he moved only a few units down from where he had been living) it apparently had not been updated **everywhere it needed it be**, which confused him and surprised him. (After all, when one is dealing with a single corporation, shouldn't one's mailing address need not be updated more than once?) I'm sure he wondered that. With our bank, however, address changes must be updated in the customer's affiliate for deposit account statements, and then **again** in our Bancorp headquarter's database for credit or debit card mailings. Often new employees don't realize this and think the job is done after simply updating the customer's local address record.*

Being that it involved a credit card the customer was particularly upset. You see, the new owner of the condo he had lived in set the envelope on top of the mailboxes, where a friend in the same complex, who knew where the doctor now lived, fortunately noticed it and delivered it to him!

I apologized to the customer for the mistake, took his new address, and said I would make sure it never happened again. After pulling the gentleman's address record in our local bank records, however, I discovered four customer records for him, with two different but extremely close social security numbers. In the Bancorp records, believe it or not, I found six records in variations of his name, again with two social security numbers. I had no idea which social was correct so I had to call him to verify it, exposing yet another bank error to him. He gave me the correct social. I told him I would take care of combining all the various records into one per affiliate. He thanked me more than once for the "good follow up."

He stopped in the bank the other day while I was busy at my office manager's desk. It had been about a month since the problem had been solved. On his way out the door he stopped at

the desk to introduce himself again and to thank me yet again
for doing such a good job. I told him that's what I was there for.
   Mike Ferrell, New Accounts Representative,
   Columbus, Ohio

Customers are so grateful when a bank employee not only tells them they will handle their problem but they actually FIX the problem! You can bet that customer will always come to Mike the next time he has a problem because Mike is the bank to that customer.

Robot Service

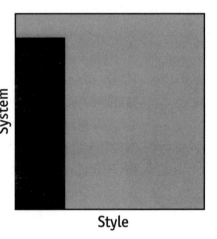

With this type of service, your bank does really well with the *system* dimension only. You have rules and regulations for everything. You have comprehensive procedures. You have policies and fees for just about everything. But you don't really care about me as a customer. You are rude, apathetic, and indifferent when it comes to how you deliver your service, i.e. *style.*

   From a closed account survey: "I felt that my account meant nothing to ABC Bank. I felt service and tellers were rude, unwilling to assist myself and my fiancé, and I plan on never returning."

As a result, here's what your customers might be saying about your bank's service: "Gosh, they just don't bend the rules." "You're inflexible." "You don't care about me as an individual." "You are indifferent, and you just give me a short, quick response and act like I'm in the way."

Here's the bottom-line message when you provide **Robot** Service:

"Don't hide behind our "policies and procedures." Clearly explain the reasons behind the situation. Offer alternatives. Ask the customer for their suggestions for resolving issues. You would be surprised that the customer's request can often easily be met!"

Roger Furrer, Commercial Banking Senior Vice President,
Western Ohio Fifth Third Bank

"You are an account number and we're here to get you through the line as fast as we can." You are an account number. Perhaps you are a loan number. Either way, you are simply a number and our job is to process you. No personal touch, no name recognition, no personal service. We are robots and our job it to get you through our line as quickly as possible.

The most relatable example that I have come up with is the U.S. Postal Service. I believe that the U.S. mail service is accurate and, for the most part, reliable. But I've never been to a post office where they've greeted me with a smile and said, "Welcome to the United States Postal Service. How may I be of assistance to you?" *(style)* No, my experience has been closer to a gruff and unfriendly: "NEXT!" Or "Don't cross that yellow line until I've called you." The Postal Service has not really emphasized the *style* side of how they deliver customer service until eight or ten years ago. Suddenly, I noticed that they had little customer comment cards in the lobby area and I thought, "Hmm, that's unusual. They have mediocre customer service at best. Why do they suddenly care what I think about them as a customer?" Then it suddenly struck me: Federal Express…UPS. When they had little or no competition, they could treat me like a robot because I didn't have other options. Although most letters still only go through the U.S. Postal Service, their package business has dropped dramatically due to competition. What would happen to your bank's service if you had little or no competition? The reality for banks is that you have enormous competition for almost every customer that you have.

Customers Desire Personal, Not Robot, Service

"I came to the United States from South Africa in September 1987 when all banks were extremely goosy due to the Savings & Loan scandal. I arrived to turn around a com-

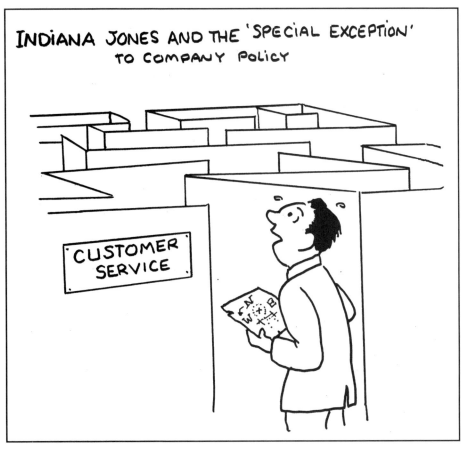

INDIANA JONES AND THE 'SPECIAL EXCEPTION' TO COMPANY POLICY

CUSTOMER SERVICE

pletely insolvent major travel group, which owed Oaks Bank $800,000. The president of Oaks Bank at the time, Lex Johnston, trusted me, as a South African CPA, to turn around the ailing group. He and Oaks Bank helped me with the recovery of the group's financial situation by loaning me money - sometimes up to $250,000 - each week to pay the airlines, knowing full well that I would keep my word and repay on time. We developed the utmost respect for each other, and he gave me excellent advice.

A few years later, Lex mailed me a letter, which I still have at home, that read, 'All the notes that were owing have been repaid, which is a tribute to your managerial ability.' I certain-

ly could not have done that on my own, and it wasn't just Lex, but everyone in the bank who trusted me as their client. Their actions showed they regarded me as a client for the long-term.

I left the travel company nine years ago after returning it to profitability and suffering an injustice. I came to see Max, the chairman of the bank, who told me to dry up the tears and start again. I followed his excellent advice, and have continued banking with the bank. If any of my clients' need a reference, I tell them to call Oaks Bank, since they know me and all my financial habits, which are very conservative. I have always kept the people at Oaks Bank fully informed of my financial plans, and give them good reason when I need their temporary

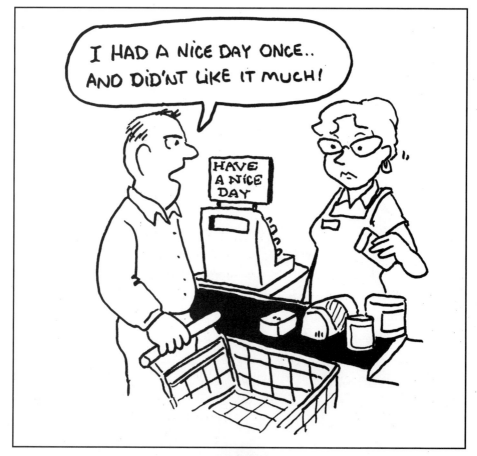

assistance. This is the epitome of personal relationship banking, where you're not a number, but an esteemed client, in the true sense of the word."
　　Michael, Dallas, TX

People DON'T want fast, accurate service with no personal touch. Customers get tired of being treated like a number. We want a personal touch. We want you to remember our name and to build a relationship with us so we can come back and refer others to you.

Is your bank's system in place to service your customers, or is it in place to make it easier for your bank? How difficult is it to get through your system? As your customer, do I get a quick response to the phone calls that I make to you? Or do I have to fill out 14 pieces of paperwork or make 13 phone calls just to get something done as a customer? Oftentimes, banks have systems in place to make it convenient for the bank. This can make it very difficult to get a job done right for a customer.

Beware of Robots

I don't know if you've been to K-Mart recently, but what do they say upon your exit from the store? They are required to say: "Thank you for shopping at K-Mart." In fact TYFSAK is posted on every single cash register as a reminder to the clerks. I don't know about your personal experience, but I've never really felt appreciated for shopping at K-Mart. I usually leave in a rush, in a hurry and get out of their way. But they do say the "right" words.

Now, for those of you whose bank uses a mystery shop program, I find some tellers are resistant to the fact that you must use certain phrases in order to score a 100 percent. I believe that mystery shop services have their place and tend to reward good service. However, I think it's more important HOW you say things than WHAT you say specifically (we address this much more in the Rapport Book). If you become robotic in your responses to customers, you will be losing that personal touch feel that is important to many of your customers. Use your bank's phrases, but please do so with your own personality.

Clueless Service

In this type of service, you just smile, smile, smile — but clearly you have no idea what you're doing. Your bank's *system* has very evident problems and everything seems to go wrong, but you are so nice about these problems. Here are some ways your customers might describe this service: "They have great service, but

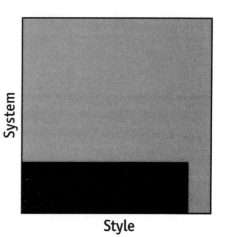

Style

they just don't know anything about their products." "That bank is friendly but boy, do they hire stupid tellers." "They have such sloppy ways of doing things."

Here's the bottom-line message for the clueless service providers: *"Do we look like we know what we're doing?"* This is what I call Alice in Wonderland service. Alice went to Wonderland. It was so much fun. They had cookies and punch and food and they smiled. They played games, they had such a good time, but she didn't know if she could get out alive.

You know what? You are dealing with your customer's money and that's nothing to joke about. I don't care how warm and friendly you are, you must still do things correctly for your customers. You can do all those wonderful personal *style* things, but if you mess up your customer's account, you are talking about how your customer supports their life and family.

Here's an important question for you to consider: Have you earned the right to get ALL of your customer's banking business – their home mortgage, a home equity loan, car loan, VISA, investments, annuity, and CDs? Think about it. Your bank has many products and services, but every one of your customers is looking at how well you do the basics before they give you any other part of their business. This has very little to do with cross-selling and everything to do with the kind of professional service and knowledge I receive from you and how well your bank handles my current business with you. Do you know your products and my situation so that I can trust you to recommend products that would help ME?

"Upon graduation from the State University, I began looking for a better bank within which to invest my money. I then

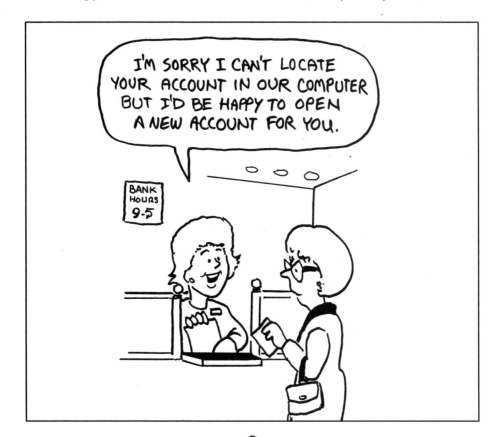

went to the ABC Bank at such-and-such a location. I stated that I wanted to close my savings account. I was never asked why I was unsatisfied with my service at ABC Bank. The woman who assisted me closed out my account and gave me a check for everything in my savings account up to the interest I had earned that day.

Within five days, I received a letter in the mail from ABC Bank stating my savings account had been overdrawn by the exact same amount I had been given in interest when I closed out my account. I immediately went to a second ABC Bank location with documentation that I had not overdrawn but I was actually due the money that I was given. After speaking with a woman who had no idea what I was talking about and couldn't follow my line of reasoning, another lady who happened to overhear our conversation came over and stated she knew exactly what happened. It happens all the time.

Enraged, I left the bank. Why, I asked, if the situation happened even once before let alone all the time, was it continuing to occur? Why hadn't someone fixed the error so I would not have to deal with the stress of receiving a letter that said I was overdrawn and accumulating charges on an account that I had closed five days earlier?

Finally, I went to a third ABC Bank location to close my checking account. Once again, I was not asked why I was moving my account to another bank. I asked the gentleman who was helping me if he would like to know, and his response was to stare at me without speaking. The gentleman began counting out money for me when I asked for a check. He informed that I would have to pay for this check, even though I was given a check by the first branch with no questions asked. The gentleman refused to write a check for me and I walked out of the bank with a rather large sum of money in my pocket making me feel very uncomfortable."

Why did the student who sent this letter not consider ABC Bank for his investments? Why were there so many inconsistencies in the three different branches that this student went to? You can be as nice as you want, but if your bank doesn't have *systems* in place that are consistently applied at all locations, your customers and therefore the bank will run into problems.

Customer Service that Creates Loyalty

The final type of customer service is the only kind of service that creates loyal customers. You are doing everything right — You have the personal *style* dimension going for you and your *system* dimension works well so that your bank rarely makes errors. Customers love you and they want to refer business to you.

Style

Here's how customers might describe this type of service: "Wow! What friendly and competent service they provide. I trust my bank." I'm going to tell my business colleagues about their great products and service. My associates can't go wrong with this bank" "My bank's tellers are knowledgeable and they are able to help me with what I need." "I love their friendliness." "They did what it took to solve my problem and I only had to call once!" "They understand my needs and empathized with my situation."

Here's the bottom-line message: *"We deliver because we care!"*

> *"Just a note to applaud the ladies of Fifth Third Bank in Hilliard, Ohio. There is usually a small staff but they are strong competent women. Each seems unnerved by a line that*

may form. Each customer has a personal touch/feel when it's one's turn. They are the only reason we continue at Fifth Third Bank.

They were always helpful getting money to the correct for our then college student daughter when we often didn't have her account number. They have been great with my 76-year-old mother sending money from California. She has closed all her previous accounts from Columbus except our Hilliard branch. Several of the employees have sort out her questions by phone. God love them. During the death of oldest son in July, three of the ladies came to the calling hours to comfort us."

The Customer Service Representatives at this bank went above and beyond most of the expectations we would have of a bank. They not only delivered great *service* to this family (with the grandmother and college student), they cared enough to express sympathy for their customer's loss.

The best analogy I've come up with to represent this type of service is Rudolph-the-red-nosed-reindeer. Do you remember how many reindeer in all there were? There were nine. Now, without singing the song in your head, can you name all nine reindeer? Most of us cannot remember all nine reindeer. Yet, if I asked a typical person to name a reindeer, whom would they name? Rudolph.

Would you agree with me that all the reindeer had all the same technical or *system* ability to fly through the night? Yes. There was one major difference between Rudolph and the other reindeer: Rudolph had a "can-do" *style*. You see, Santa Claus had a problem. As the story goes, Santa came to the reindeer on Christmas Eve during a huge snowstorm. A major snowstorm. All the other reindeer were not interested in getting out in the bitter snowstorm that night to deliver presents to the children.

This was a huge problem for Santa Claus. He came to the barn and said to Rudolph, "Rudolph, I have a problem. Would you be willing to

lead the sleigh tonight?" And Rudolph
said, "You have a problem? Great! I'll do
what you need me to do. I'll lead the
sleigh tonight." Rudolph is a reindeer
with a can-do *style* and attitude. The
other reindeer said, "I don't wanna fly, I
don't wanna do this." In contrast,
Rudolph said, "You have a problem?
Great! I'll handle it."

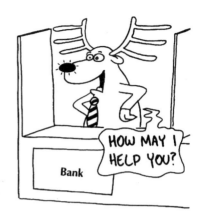

Let's compare that analogy to banks.
Would you agree with me that all of the banking competitors in your
town have basically the same *systems* you have? Same products? Same
services? Pretty much the same fees? Same interest rates? Really, if you
think about it, there is very little difference between you and every single bank when it comes to the *system* side of service. The difference has
to be that the people who work in your bank need to have the Rudolph
can-do *style* of attitude. If I come to your city and ask people on the street:
Name the best bank in town – what would they say? "Hmmm — best
bank? Let me think about that." If your bank is not the first one that
comes to mind, you are not winning the competitive game. There is
tremendous competition out there with all the other banks that are trying
to win YOUR customers over to their bank. You have a huge opportunity as a bank in your city to grow your bank's business by leaps and
bounds if you are Rudolph to every single customer who comes in.

Rudolph Service

"I was in real estate when I started banking at Oaks. I bor-
rowed money from the bank after meeting Max Wells over
lunch, and shortly thereafter, real estate went to hell in a hand
basket. I had three partners, two who went bankrupt. My other
partner and I went in to the bank and recapitalized the loan

with personal guarantees, including my old truck, and promised to get them taken care of. Oaks didn't sue, take anything away, or cause any greater harm, but accepted the terms, and let me pay them back accordingly.

"While we were recovering, my wife and I would have to stop by the bank every day to check our balance and verify which checks we could actually write and cover. In those days, you couldn't do that on the phone or Internet, and my wife had two young children, so the bank staff would hand-write the balance and deliver it to her in the car.

"One thing that is unique about banking at Oaks is not only that a person answers the phone, but also that that person, Barbara, has been there for 10 years; Kyle, the Executive Vice President, has been there for 15 years; his assistant Renee has been there for more than 10, and of course Max, has been there since he and Lex founded the bank in 1985. They seem to find a way to always do something, acting as deal makers rather than deal killers."

Robert, Denton, TX

Oaks Bank could have easily gotten rid of this "bad" customer – after all, the bank could lose a lot of money. Or, they could choose to work with the customer and gain a customer for life. They chose to do the later and be a 'Rudolph' to save the night for their customer.

To be Rudolph, you must "own" each and every customer's problem whether they are standing in front of you or they call you on the phone. You must have a great, can-do attitude and be committed and knowledgeable about your bank's products and services.

Do You Have the RIGHT Stuff?

Many customers will judge their bank's effectiveness based on their first problem experience. Are you a "one and done" bank? The customer contacts "one" person and that person handles the problem and it's "done" – taken care of. That's the ideal scenario for your customers and one that creates customer loyalty.

Here are some key strategies to implement so that you can be a "one and done" employee. We'll use the acronym R.I.G.H.T. to see if you have the right stuff:

Rapport:

Build Rapport by acknowledging the customer as soon as they enter your banking center. This also has another benefit: Do you realize that most bank security officers will tell you that the single greatest action you can take to prevent a robbery is to acknowledge people when they come into your branch?

Use your customer's name during each interaction. It's simple and easy to get your customer's name off of their account information or deposit slip – yet it makes all the difference for your customer's perception of your service! Can you tell me the eye color of each of your customers? If not, you probably didn't really make a connection with them. Read the Banking Secrets Rapport book for many more ideas on this topic.

When a customer comes to you with a problem, you need to listen to them. Take notes. Figure out exactly what the problem is and solve it. If you can solve their problem quickly and to their complete satisfaction 80 percent of the time, they'll become happy and loyal customers.

When someone comes into your banking center or calls you on the phone, do you listen long enough to figure out what their *real* problem is? Many times customers will call their branch first even if they know you probably can't answer their questions. Remember – YOU are the bank to them. Do you ask enough questions to help determine the correct department that will be able to help them? Please don't just transfer them to any department to simply get rid of the "problem."

Inform Customers What You Can Do To Help Them

The "I" in RIGHT stuff means to inform customers what you can do to help them. Be polite. Hear all your customer has to say without interrupting them. If they are on the phone, give them oral feedback that says you are listening: "Uh-huh." "Okay. Let me summarize what you've said so far." Your purpose is to solve the problem on their first call. Don't force them to make multiple phone calls or trips because you didn't fix their problem. You goal is to be done with it. Ask questions if you need to. Restate the problem to the customer to make sure that you really understand their problem. At the end of your conversation with the customer, give them your name and phone number —"Ms. Customer —let me know if there is anything else I can do for you." That's informing customers what you can do to help them.

Know the bank's products and services. The weakest link in any customer service department is lack of knowledge. Does your bank have an internal phone directory that is specific to the types of phone calls that come in so that you know where and to whom to transfer the customer? If not, make that suggestion to your training or marketing department.

> *"Anyone can make a mistake. But a mistake with three separate cover-ups, unreturned phone calls, an attempt to defraud $40, and stories that change weekly have lost you a lifetime customer.*

" The key to handling a "difficult" customer is to never lose sight of the fact that they are a customer. Love 'em or hate 'em, they keep the lights on."

Douglas Singer, Senior Vice President Branch Network Sales,
National City Bank

> *I read somewhere that banks typically expect to pay more*
> *than $100 to attract new credit card customers. In retrospect,*
> *you lost one in an attempt to gouge $40; that's bad math.*
> *Additionally, my husband and I have thousands of dollars in*
> *both checking and savings accounts with your bank involving*
> *our rental properties and personal business. I will scout other*
> *banks next week."*
> *Barbara, Columbus, Ohio*

Why didn't someone inform Barbara how s/he would fix her problem? Each employee she contacted made an excuse or passed Barbara's problem on to the next employee. In losing Barbara's credit card business, they also lost her checking account, savings account, and mortgage loan business — a huge price for that bank to pay for poor customer service. It only takes one person to own and fix a customer's problem — will that person be you?

Get the Problem Solved

This is really about problem ownership. Remember Rudolph? When Santa Claus had a problem and asked for Rudolph's help, Rudolph didn't hesitate to be a leader. Don't argue with the customer. I dislike the comment "the customer is always right," because the customer is *not* always right. But the point is, the customer is still the customer. I don't care if they are not right. When you try to show that they are wrong, you just enflame them.

You need to make the phone calls for the customer. If it's the customer's third time that they've been transferred, wouldn't it make sense for you to say, "Let me find out exactly who you need to speak to," and spend a couple of extra minutes with the person to make sure you know where they can get their problem solved? The more you can own your customers' problem, the better off they and your bank will be.

Ask the customer how you can make it right. Apologize if the customer thinks the bank made a mistake. The quickest way to get a customer over their anger is to apologize – why would they continue yelling at you when you just admitted that you (or the bank) was wrong?

I had banked at a local establishment for a number of years when I decided to get a cash advance on my credit card for a vacation. When I got to the teller and asked her assistance, she proceeded to tell me that I had to go to "my bank" in order to get a cash advance. I assured her that this was my bank. Well, we went round and round about me having to go to "my bank" for the cash advance and that I was at my bank when finally she told me that I had to go to the bank that the credit card was issued from to get the cash advance.

Needless to say I was dumbfounded because the credit card was issued from a bank in Ohio and I live in Missouri. When I explained this to the teller, she raised her hands (like she was being robbed), took three steps backward and said very loudly " I cannot help you". OK, now I was embarrassed because everyone, including the security guard was staring at me. I left without my cash advance.

What makes this story even more frightening is that a year or so later I was robbed at the ATM on the outside of the bank. I wanted to remove all of my money from the bank because I did not feel comfortable going to that bank any longer so I went with a friend one afternoon to close my account. When I explained that I wanted to close the account but knew that there would be an automatic withdrawal soon for a payment and that I wanted to leave that exact amount in the account to cover the payment then consider the account closed, the teller stated that it couldn't be done. I explained that I had been robbed and did not feel comfortable returning but she would not say anything

but "I cannot help you" and yes, raised her hands as if she were being robbed and took three steps back. I asked if anyone could help and she pointed to a supervisor. I proceeded to the supervisor, explained my situation and request and you guessed it, the supervisor raised her hands, moved three steps back and said, " I cannot help you".

I left the bank very upset and still with the account open. I had to write a letter explaining the situation to close the account after the automatic withdrawal was made. To this day, my friend says that she wouldn't have believed it if she hadn't seen it for herself. The staff at this bank must have been trained to raise their hands, step back and say, "I cannot help you" in any situation that was unsolvable.

Cindy B., St. Louis, Missouri

In Cindy's situation, no one was willing to help her solve her problem. In fact, they made Cindy appear to be the problem. Keep in mind, many customer don't become a "problem" unless the bank has made a mistake in the first place.

Help The Customer Understand How You Have Solved the Problem

When you are trying to solve a problem, take the specific action necessary to solve their problem. Tell them what's going to happen next. Keep them informed throughout the problem resolution phase. If it's an account number or an address correction problem, follow-up with them and let them know how you handled their problem. Don't assume they will find out when they receive their next statement. The interesting thing about following-up is that this step is unexpected by most customers. By following up with the customer, you are showing that the customer's satisfaction is important to both you and your bank.

When I have promotional materials printed at my local Ink Well

"Own The Problem!" "Be A Rudolph!"

NAME: _____

DATE:_____TIME: _____ACCT#: _____

WORK Phone:_____HOME Phone: _____

PAGER/CELL: _____

Customer **MUST** be called back! Date/Time of promised call-back:_____

———————————— DUTY TO BE DONE ————————————

_____ **CHANGE ADDR/PH#** (Joint owners? Other affiliates?)

Address:_____

Home: _____Work: _____

City/St/Zip: _____

_____ **CHECK ORDER** (Get a phone number if the order is not placed in the customer's presence)

Style: Same / Other   Starting check #: _____   # of boxes: _____   Mail to branch? (Y / N)

Personalization changes (see address changes above):_____

_____

"I'VE GOT A PROBLEM!" :

_____

_____

_____

_____

_____

FOLLOW-UP / PROBLEM RESOLUTION LOG:

PH #_____

DATE CALLED _____SPOKE TO _____

DETAILS AND CURRENT STATUS _____

_____

PH #_____

DATE CALLED _____SPOKE TO _____

DETAILS AND CURRENT STATUS _____

_____

PH #_____

DATE CALLED _____SPOKE TO _____

DETAILS AND CURRENT STATUS _____

_____

_____

store, they always call me up. "Patti, how was your order? Were there any problems with it? Is there anything we can do to help you?" I know I can expect that follow-up phone call. I have never had a problem with my print job, but I always think to myself, "Wow, that was nice. They really value my business."

A special thanks to Mike Ferrell of Fifth Third Bank in Columbus, Ohio, who developed this form to keep track of his customer problems. Go to www.bankingsecrets.com for a downloadable version of this form that you can adapt for your own situation.

Take Complaints as a Gift

Only when we begin viewing complaints as a gift and invitation for improvement from our customer will we be on the road to earning loyalty from our customers. How well do you handle complaints and criticism from your customers?

Here's a brief self-assessment to see how you currently handle complaints and criticism in your job at the bank. I've included both internal and external customer examples. Place a "plus" (+) by those situations that you feel you handle appropriately, a "minus" (-) by those situations you avoid handling, and a "zero" (0) by those you handle but not well.

____ You are trying to reach an internal department at your bank's corporate office. Your branch customer is getting agitated because he has a simple problem that is taking much longer to fix than was expected.

____ Your supervisor criticizes your job performance.

____ A customer on the phone is upset about the fees that have changed on his checking account. You are the third person he has been transferred to.

____ You hear from a colleague that your supervisor is upset about a comment you made yesterday.

____ A customer criticizes you for something you know you didn't do.

____ A customer standing in front of you is very upset about a letter they received from your bank saying their car payments are behind and that the bank will come and seize their car. They have canceled checks proving they have made all payments.

____ Things haven't been going well for you lately and you are feeling down, a co-worker criticizes you for your "bad attitude".

____ A customer ordered express checks 5 days ago and still hasn't received them.

____ This is the third time this month that your customer is checking on a correction you submitted over three weeks ago.

____ A recently acquired banking customer is frustrated with the fact that your bank is not "on-line."

____ A customer on the phone starts yelling at you for something for which you are not responsible.

What other scenarios have occurred at work in which you have been criticized and/or been complained to and you would like to deal more effectively?

_____

_____

_____

_____

We have no control over how a customer complains to us. We do, however, have total control over how we *react* to their complaint. Naturally, we will react to a customer's complaint or criticism one of two ways: (1) We become passive or a silent victim, or (2) We become aggressive and counter-attack our critic.

Let's look at the pros and cons of these two instinctive responses. When we counterattack our critic, we often do so with sarcasm, put downs, or digs. I'm often amazed at how often people attend my "Dealing with Difficult People" workshops merely looking for the quick put downs or counterattacks. In fact, sometimes our one-liners are real "zingers" and, if we have an audience, we may get a big laugh out of them. Someone once told me that the Greek translation for sarcasm is "tear flesh." It is an excellent word picture for the damage sarcasm brings to the criticized.

Comedians and cartoonists use sarcasm often to create humor. For example: "My wife started to diet when she went from a size 9 to a size tent." Although it's a funny statement, it cuts to the heart of the person being put down.

The downside of being aggressive or counterattacking is obvious. You have not helped to build a relationship, but instead have resorted to putting your critic down. This does not promote a climate in which you can comfortably continue to talk with your critic, nor your critic with you. It certainly will make your customers angry. When it comes to dealing with customers, counterattacking has no place.

When we counterattack an aggressive customer who is complaining to us, we may think we are not affecting that person. However, our customer may not be as thick-skinned as we might have imagined. Often, critical people are as insecure as people who behave passively.

The silent victim or passive approach is no more helpful. If you say nothing or accept the criticism as valid before assessing it, you will appear to have little self-confidence and may lose the respect of others and yourself! Secondly, you may not truly understand what the critic intended by the criticism unless you take time to assess the criticism.

The point is to not automatically assume your critic is right nor to automatically change your behavior. A far better approach to handling criticism is to be aware that criticism is "just criticism" and then move quickly to assessing its merit.

If you have an internal customer (i.e. supervisor or co-worker) who is criticizing you, take time to assess how the criticism was delivered, the intent of the critic, and how valid you believe the criticism to be. It is at this point that you may want to ask yourself a couple of questions to determine whether or not the criticism is valid:

1. Do I hear the same criticism from other customers?

2. Does the critic know a great deal about this topic?

3. Are the critic's expectations reasonable?

4. Is the criticism really about me? (or is the critic merely having a

bad day or upset about something else)

5.   How important is it for me to respond immediately in this situation?

Watch also for the nonverbal behavior of your critic. You may be able to determine the intensity of his or her feelings and how open he or she will be to the action you decide to take.

Let's examine some action strategies for dealing assertively with the complaints or criticism your customers may give you.

Being Gracious with Complaints

If we think of complaints as gifts, it will allow us to remain confident and cool. An assertive approach permits a "win-win" attitude in which you allow your critic to have an opinion while maintaining your own. Manuel J. Smith, author of *When I Say No, I Feel Guilty*, introduces three assertive techniques that I have adapted. These techniques have proven to be invaluable in helping assess and evaluate what action to take when a customer complains to you. Keep in mind, your customer's complaint can be a gift in that the bank can become better if you listen, respond and solve the complaint.

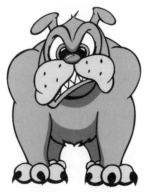

If you're dog-tired at night, maybe it's because you growled all day."

The three techniques are: Fogging, Admitting the Truth, and Asking for Specific Feedback. We will review each of these techniques by examining the situation and types of criticism with which they are most effective.

Who Asked You for Your Opinion Anyway?
Dealing with Unjustified Criticism and Advice

The first criticism technique is ideal for dealing with *unjustified criticism*. More often than not this type of criticism comes from your internal customers – your co-workers, boss, and/or employees from other departments. When you receive this type of criticism, force yourself to avoid the natural reaction of counter criticizing or counter manipulating your critic. We often receive this type of criticism in the form of advice — often both unwarranted and unasked for!

The first thing we must do when someone criticizes us invalidly or unjustifiably is to set up a psychological barrier that protects us from taking the criticism personally. One of the foundations for handling complaints effectively is self-confidence and high self-esteem. If we believe in ourselves, in our abilities, skills, and knowledge, then the complaint is much less threatening, and we tend to take it less personally. The bottom line is that we must choose to let the complaint have no devastating impact and not impact how we treat the next customer.

An example might be a co-worker who overhears your comments to a customer and says, "Boy, I just overheard what you said to your last customer. I'm not sure that is the approach you should have taken."

Naturally, there are two ways to respond to your co-worker: (1) Mumble and/or admit that we were wrong (a passive approach); or (2) we could tell the co-worker where they could go with their opinion (the aggressive route). A far better approach would be to utilize the assertive

FOGGING technique, which calmly acknowledges that there MAY be some truth in the criticism.

What fogging does is that it allows you to receive the criticism without becoming anxious or defensive. It allows you to be the final judge of what to do about it. You become a listener instead of a reader of minds. The result is like a fog bank: you are unaffected by manipulative, unjustified criticism. After awhile, your co-worker finds it's no fun to throw things at you.

For the previous criticism from your co-worker, you could fog them by saying, "Perhaps I could've responded to the customer differently." You don't say to your co-worker that they are absolutely right and you don't tell them they are absolutely wrong. You merely agree that there may be <u>some</u> truth in the statement. Other potential fogging responses might begin with:

You might be right about . . .

You could be right about . . .

What you say makes sense . . .

One of the criticisms my mom likes to give me is the need for me to take more vitamins. Because I travel with my speaking business, have contact with lots of people, and have two young boys at home, I do occasionally get a cold during the winter. My Mom's advice to me goes something like this, "Patti, I think you should take more vitamin C. You know just the other day I read in *Prevention* magazine that if you take 20,000 mega doses of vitamin C per day, you'll have 60% less colds a year."

Admittedly, my natural response to my mother would go something like this . . . "Oh mother, you know vitamin C has little to do with the common cold." Well, you can imagine what would happen as a result . . . we would have a major argument about vitamin C and the pros and cons of taking it. Is this worth arguing about? No.

So what I do instead is to use a Fogging Response like . . . "Maybe I should take more vitamin C." And then I change the subject. My mom isn't sure what just happened. Did I agree with her? or disagree? It's like being surrounded by a fog bank. I move on before the fog has a chance to clear. Meanwhile, after the conversation, I can decide whether or not I want to take vitamin C.

It's important to note that often unjustified criticism is expressed in broad, general terms, which are unrealistic, untrue, and often spoken out of anger. When encountering criticism, watch out for words like "always," "never," "all the time," and "every time." Many times, this indicates the criticism is unjustified and a fogging response is appropriate.

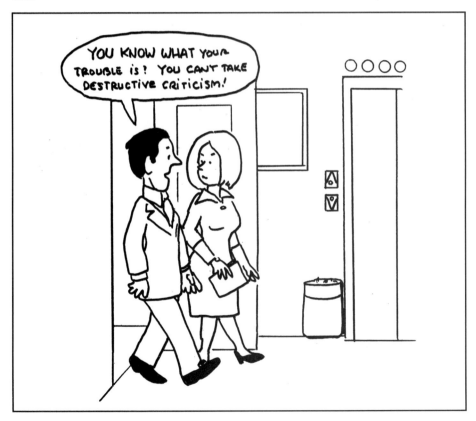

Let's look at an actual customer situation in which the teller did NOT respond in a way that solved the customer's problem but merely angered her:

> *"As is generally my custom on payday, I came to your bank to cash my check and pay some bills. I used the drive-through window in order to save some time. When I received the container from the teller, I did not leave the area until I had counted what should have been my receipt and my money.*
>
> *I immediately noticed that I had been shorted $100. When I attempted to report this to the teller, she insisted that she had provided me with all that was coming to me. I asked for her supervisor and decided to enter the bank.*
>
> *The more I tried to reason with her, the more adamant and boisterous she became. She and the supervisor seemed to get louder and more persistent and it was extremely publicly humiliating. Are banking people so exalted that they cannot make mistakes?*
>
> *I was told that if I wanted them to investigate that I would have to return at 7:00 p.m. after the bank closed. This did not seem reasonable to me, as it was my money that they were keeping and accusing me of lying about. I refused to leave without my money. The attention of all those in the bank were on me. I was being treated as though I were a criminal.*
>
> [They counted the money and found that they had indeed shorted the customer $100]... *the supervisor leaned over toward me and in whispered tones said, "We have found your money." I have never, in the many years that I have been banking at that branch, been treated in such a manner. The treatment was abhorrent!*
>
> *There is no reason or excuse to treat any other customer, or me whatever our race, as if we were liars or hardened criminals. I take faith in the fact that this will not happen again . . . I am*

*not unaware that we are all human and as such, we are subject
to make mistakes but this does not imply that we should be less
than civil to one another."*

How much better could this situation have been handled if the CSR
would have said immediately to the customer, "Perhaps, I did miscount
your cash. Would you mind coming in to the bank and I will immediately count my drawer and check for you?" Never assume your customer is wrong until the facts confirm it. Always veer on the side of the
customer until proven differently.

An easy mistake for people to make with the fogging technique is to
"Yes, but . . ." That is, to make a good fogging statement and then add on
the reasons why they did what they did. Take the previous example.

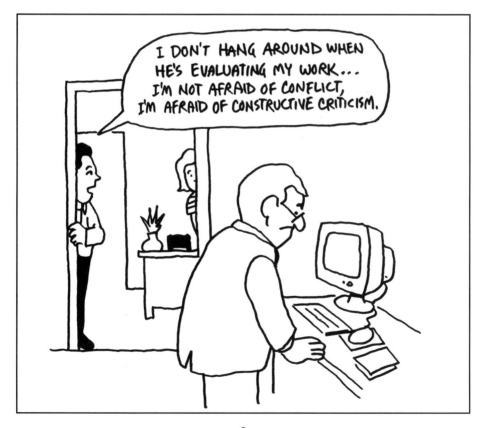

"Yes, perhaps I did miscount your money, <u>but</u> we are always so short-staffed and busy it's nearly impossible to have 100% accuracy." A good fogging statement uses active listening skills to paraphrase the criticism but doesn't add any excuses or rationalizations.

One of the greatest benefits to fogging is that it forces you to *listen* to your customer/co-worker/supervisor instead of automatically reacting to his/her comments. The result is that you are learning more about the problem in the process. Secondly, after you have handled the situation, you can decide whether or not the complaint has any merit and whether or not you want to take any action.

If you choose NOT to use the fogging technique, then you have several other options: You can grin and bear it. You can ignore it (but watch out for your nonverbal reactions, which may give away your true feelings). Or you can disagree politely. Always keep in mind that when handling unjustified criticism, you need to consider who is complaining. To what degree is the complaint a reflection of your critic's personality and motivation? Are they really trying to be helpful or do they have other motives?

Consider when using the fogging technique that there is always room for more than one opinion. Rarely is anything so black and white that it is worth arguing about. The goal of fogging is to stop the criticism. Later, you can decide whether or not to do something about the situation that provoked the criticism in the first place.

"Sorry" is the Hardest Word to Say: Dealing with Valid Complaints

The second technique of ADMITTING THE TRUTH is very effective when handling *valid complaints*. That is, accept your mistakes and faults without <u>over</u> apologizing for them. Too often when we make a mistake we try and cover it up. Perhaps the root of cover-ups lie in our childhood of getting "caught" and our fear of punishment. But in reality, the best thing we can do is to admit we made a mistake and move on into the future.

When you admit the truth, it desensitizes you to criticism from yourself or others. It allows you to recognize mistakes as mistakes. The result is that once you accept your mistakes, you can move forward, rather than becoming bogged down in depression and self-criticism. It also helps extinguish the complaint.

In the Spring 2002 issue of the Gallup Management Journal*, they reported one case where a major bank was still suffering from damaged customer relationships 14 months after a spate of service problems were poorly handled. Remember, when we have poor customer service, we take every opportunity we have to share that information with others. Negative word-of-mouth problems do not go away quickly.

Here's the good news about complaints that are handled well. When Gallup surveyed retail banking customers, only 26% of those who had not recently had a problem considered themselves extremely satisfied with the bank versus 51% who had experienced a problem but were extremely satisfied with the way it was handled. Gallup states, "If the company owns the problem, apologizes and undertakes a remedy, the customer's perceptions are validated and his value to the company is confirmed."

Potential replies to valid complaints might include: "You're right, we didn't get the correct address on your account. I'm very sorry. I'm correcting it in our computer right now." "You're right. Your balance is not correct in our system. Let me correct that for you and print a receipt out for you." The key here is to not *over* apologize. If you miscounted the cash that is owed to your customer, you wouldn't say, "You are right. I

* Reprinted with permission from The Gallup Management Journal ©2002, all rights reserved. The complete article can be found at: http://www.gallupjournal.com/GMJarchive/ issue5/2002315g.asp

miscounted your cash. Whew! You are fourth customer today that I counted the cash for." Too much information! I really don't want to know how many errors you have made with other customers in that I'm beginning to lose my confidence in you. In the miscounted cash scenario, simply say, "You were right, I did miscount your cash. I'm very sorry and apologize for any inconvenience." Be sincere and sound like you are truly sorry.

Additional things to think about when responding to valid complaints include:

- Focus on the present, not the past.

- Accept responsibility for the mistake but don't indulge in self put-downs.

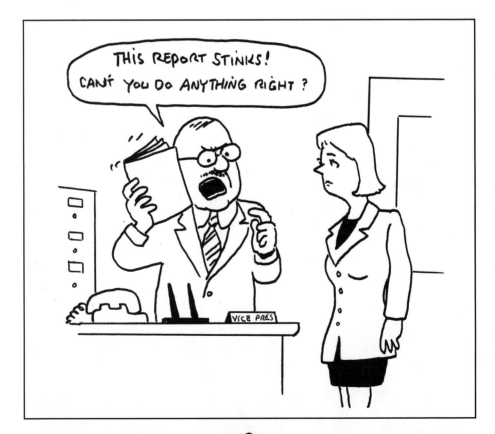

- Avoid denying, counter-criticizing, over-apologizing or over-compensating. You need to agree with the specifics of your mistake.

- Assess if there is anything you can do NOW about the situation and work to negotiate a compromise.

> *"I received checks from the bank with the incorrect account number. When I tried to find out why they returned the checks "insufficient funds", I was told that my account was closed. It took me 20 phone calls; three trips to the bank branch, and one to the main branch to find the bank put the wrong number on my checks.*
>
> *After this fiasco which was entirely the bank's fault, the bank refused to help me remedy the issues of late charges and returned check fees until I threatened to bring in an attorney to discuss this with the bank. This was not customer service! Obviously, I took my money out of that bank and now bank with someone who cares about me as a customer."*
>
> *June, Cleveland, Ohio*

A Customer's Valid Criticism

How you respond to a customer's criticism of you and your bank will probably spell the difference between them leaving your bank or remaining as a customer. Twenty phone calls and four trips to the bank is totally unacceptable when it comes to service! This problem should have been handled over the phone or at the first visit. This bank obviously does not have employees who were willing to own the problem and get it fixed. The result? Another lost customer.

Just What Do You Mean by That?
Dealing with Vague Complaints

The last type of criticism comes in the form of *vague complaints.* This is sometimes the most difficult and frustrating type of complaint you will get. In these cases, it is important to REQUEST SPECIFIC FEED-BACK. You want to prompt criticism by listening to your customer and asking questions. With the use of questions, you can begin focusing on the future instead of dwelling on the past. It moves you directly into taking action to resolve the potential problem and forces the customer to look at potential solutions instead of belaboring your failure. Also, it enlists the customer to be on your side.

Requesting specific feedback helps you to gain information you can use. As well, you exhaust your customer's complaints and often, uncover the customer's true feelings and discover common ground. The result is that you break the manipulative cycle of criticism by improving understanding and communication. Some examples include:

- What did we specifically do that was a problem? . . .

- I'm not sure I'm clear about what your perception of the problem is. Could you please give me an example?

Each of these questions will force the customer to be clearer, more precise, and will enable you to change your behavior to more effective-ly meet their expectations or needs. A sports player cannot excel with-out a coach's clear and specific instructions on what to do to improve, nor can we improve our "game" without clear feedback from our customers.

The whole idea behind this technique is to reduce the vague criticism to manageable, behavioral terms. You want to prompt your customer to be specific. Don't become defensive, counter-critical or immediately deny the criticism. Instead, try to be genuine in your desire to receive information. It may even be helpful to repeat back or paraphrase your understanding of the customer's statements.

The basic skills of admitting the truth and requesting specific feedback will help to extinguish the complaint and enable you assess whether or not there is anything you can do about the situation. It also moves you directly into a position where you can take steps to correct the mistake or negotiate a compromise.

Let's look at a couple of examples of vague complaints and how you might want to respond.

Customer:	*Bank Employee:*
"How come my bank account isn't making more money?"	How much were you expecting to make in interest on your savings account?
	Have you considered the other types of savings accounts our bank offers?
	With the amount of money I see in your savings account, I would recommend…
"The tellers in here used to be more friendly. Why are people not friendly anymore?"	What makes you think we are not friendly? What would like to see us do differently that would make you more comfortable?

It is critical when asking a customer who is vaguely criticizing the bank or you to make sure that you use a neutral tone of voice and body language. It's not only the words you use but also how you say them that makes all the difference in the world in how your questions will be received. Always be genuine.

The bottom line in handling criticism and complaints is that a true professional learns how to build a firm foundation out of the bricks that others throw at them. That is what handling complaints effectively can do for you . . . it can help you build a foundation of mutual respect and partnerships with your customers rather than building a barrier for protection from your customers.

Get On with Business by Getting Your Customer O.F.F. Their Problem

Your banking customers really don't want to switch banks – it's just too much hassle to do that. Instead, make it easy for your customers to do business with you. Be committed to **O**wning, **F**ixing, and **F**ollowing Through on problem situations for your customers and they will keep on coming back to you.

Keep in mind, YOU are the bank to your customers. Is that good news for your bank? Be Rudolph by being willing to lead the way in solving problems and overcoming barriers to providing exceptional customer service. Remember: the view upfront as Rudolph, the lead reindeer, far surpasses the view you will have if you are trying to catch him from behind. You can do it because you are "Great!"

FREE OFFER

For more information, to receive our free monthly e-mail tips newsletter, or to order any of our products, please contact:

The CHANGE AGENT_{SM}
1016 Woodglen Road
Westerville, Ohio 43081
Toll-free: 1-800-339-0973
Phone: 614-523-3633
Fax: 614-523-3515
E-mail: Patti@bankingsecrets.com or Jim@bankingsecrets.com
Websites: www.bankingsecrets.com and www.thechangeagent.com

If you would like to receive our free monthly e-mail tips newsletter filled with ideas on customer loyalty, change, and communication skills, sign up at either of our websites at: www.bankingsecrets.com or www.thechangeagent.com.

If you have a great story or quote to share for possible inclusion in our e-mail newsletter, website, articles, or future books in our *Banking Secrets for Customer Loyalty* book series, please send or e-mail it to Patti@bankingsecrets.com. We are always interested in real life stories on customer service and change. We also have many products and services described on our websites.

If you are looking for a dynamic and motivational keynote speaker or trainers who will deliver a highly *customized* program for your bank or association, please consider calling us to discuss your needs. Patti works with companies who are committed to changing their customer service culture and she motivates employees to get passionate about customer loyalty. She can deliver bottom-line results for your bank. It is Patti's desire as a speaker and an author to change people's perspective to produce positive results through the use of clear, easy-to-grasp ideas, compelling real-life stories delivered with word pictures, and a strong sense of humor.

Quick Order Form

Fax Orders: (614) 523-3515. Send this form.

Telephone Orders: Toll-free call 1-800-339-0973 or (614) 523-3633.
Have your credit card ready.

E-mail Orders: Jim@thechangeagent.com

Postal Orders: Destination Publications, Jim Hathaway, 1016 Woodglen Road,
Westerville, Ohio 43081-3236. USA. Telephone: 1-800-339-0973
or (614) 523-3633

*Please send the following books or products. I understand that I may return any of
them for a full refund — for any reason, no questions asked.*

Customer Loyalty Learning Resources:

Customer Loyalty Tips Booklets

Customer satisfaction is not enough in today's competitive marketplace. Your goal
must be to deliver such exceptional service that customers become loyal to you!
Discover powerful ideas that will give you the edge in pleasing today's demanding
customers (order can be combined with change booklet).

1 booklet	$ 5.00 each
2 - 249 booklets	$ 2.50 each

Rudolph Secrets for Customer Service CD Learning Program. In this highly entertain-
ing 73 minute program, Patti equips you with proven, practical 'Rudolph' Secrets for
building customer loyalty.

Retail Price: $14.95	Special Reader Price: $10

Smile-on-a-Stick™ (white and multi-cultural smiles available). For times when you just
don't have a smile of your own to give customers.

A. 1 Smile	$2.00
B. 10 Smiles	$17.95 (save 10%)
C. 100 Smiles	$165.95 (save 15%)

Change Management Learning Resources:

Untying the 'Nots' of Change Before You're Fit to be Tied book (192 pages). FREE change postcard and computer wallpaper of cartoons on CD-ROM with each book.

Retail Price: $19.95   Special Reader Price: $12.95

Tips Booklets - 93 Tips for Dealing with Work Change Change can be terrifying or empowering. It depends on whether you manage change or it manages you. Increase your productivity and energy by gaining mastery in the midst of work change. This booklet will provide you with tips to become a change agent rather than a change victim (order can be combined with customer loyalty booklet).

1 booklet	$ 5.00 each
2 - 249 booklets	$ 2.50 each

Untying the 'Nots' of Change Video Learning Program: Includes 90 minutes of video, a Leader's Guide, 10 *Untying the "Nots"* books, and the audio program.

Retail Price: $ 595.00   Special Reader Price: $ 495.00

Untying the 'Nots' of Change Before You're Fit to be Tied Audio Learning Program. 3 cassette audio tapes from Patti's enlightening program for employees on dealing with change. Almost 3 hours of information.

Retail Price: $ 34.95   Special Reader Price: $ 20

Communication Learning Resources:

Giving and Receiving Feedback book (104 pages) This newly revised edition is packed with valuable insights and suggestions for giving and receiving positive feedback effectively. Also, you'll discover the secrets to giving meaningful yet motivating criticism in a positive and professional manner. Includes exercises, tips, and a four-step guide to giving specific feedback that produces results in both your business and personal life.

Retail Price: $ 13.95

Managing Upward book (118 pages) An excellent guide if you're wishing to position yourself for upward professional mobility. This book introduces techniques for developing positive working relationship with those above you in the organization. It's not easy to "manage your boss," but the tips provided will help you handle and offer both praise and criticism.

Retail Price: $ 13.95

Please send more FREE information on:

❏ Speaking/Seminars   ❏ Coaching/Consulting

Name: _____

Address: _____

City: _____ State: _____ Zip: _____-__

Telephone: _____

E-mail Address: _____

Please send the following product(s):

Customer Loyalty Tips Booklets

      1 booklet $ 5.00 each

      2 - 249 booklets $ 2.50 each

Untying the 'Nots' of Change Before You're Fit to be Tied book
      Special Reader Price: $12.95

Tips Booklets - 93 Tips for Dealing with Work Change

      1 booklet $ 5.00 each   2 - 249 booklets $ 2.50 each

Untying the 'Nots' of Change Video Learning Program:

      Special Reader Price: $ 495.00

Untying the 'Nots' of Change Before You're Fit to be Tied Audio Learning Program.

      Special Reader Price: $ 20

Rudolph Secrets for Customer Service CD Learning Program.

      Special Reader Price: $10

Smile-on-a-Stick®

      A. 1 Smile $2.00   B. 10 Smiles $17.95 (save 10%)

      C. 100 Smile $165.95 (save 15%)

Giving and Receiving Feedback book $ 13.95

Managing Upward book $ 13.95

Sales tax: Please add 5.75% for products shipped to Ohio addresses.

Shipping: Actual shipping to be charged. E-mail or call for prices.

International: Actual shipping to be charged. E-mail or call for prices.

Payment: ❏ Check   ❏ Paypal

❏ Credit Card:# _____Expires _____
❏ Visa ❏ MasterCard ❏ American Express (AMEX)